# WHAT YOUR BODY IS TELLING YOU

## AND WHAT YOU CAN DO ABOUT IT

### DAVID ROWLAND

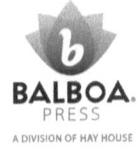

BALBOA.
PRESS

A DIVISION OF HAY HOUSE

Balboa Press books may be ordered through booksellers or by contacting:

Balboa Press
A Division of Hay House
1663 Liberty Drive
Bloomington, IN 47403
www.balboapress.com
1 (877) 407-4847

Because of the dynamic nature of the Internet, any web addresses or links contained in this book may have changed since publication and may no longer be valid. The views expressed in this work are solely those of the author and do not necessarily reflect the views of the publisher, and the publisher hereby disclaims any responsibility for them.

The author of this book does not dispense medical advice or prescribe the use of any technique as a form of treatment for physical, emotional, or medical problems without the advice of a physician, either directly or indirectly. The intent of the author is only to offer information of a general nature to help you in your quest for emotional and spiritual well-being. In the event you use any of the information in this book for yourself, which is your constitutional right, the author and the publisher assume no responsibility for your actions.

Print information available on the last page.

ISBN: 978-1-5043-7428-6 (sc)
ISBN: 978-1-5043-7453-8 (e)

Balboa Press rev. date: 02/06/2017

# Contents

# Overview

Before medicine became high tech, doctors used to take time to ask detailed questions about your symptoms. Today, laboratory tests have replaced symptom surveys. Unfortunately, blood tests for nutrients are unreliable.

The last place some deficiencies show up is in the blood. The blood strives to maintain a state of normalcy and will often do so right up to the point of death. It maintains this homeostasis at the expense of other tissues in the body. Examples: (a) blood calcium levels may be normal during osteoporosis, (b) blood levels of vitamin B-12 may be normal even when there is not enough in cerebrospinal fluid, (c) some people, under stress, produce a "mauve factor" which binds vitamin B-6 and zinc, making them unavailable to the rest of the body, (d) a vitamin B-12 deficiency can result in misleadingly high levels of folic acid, and (e) there can be enough thyroid hormone in the blood but not enough getting to the tissues that need it.

Symptom surveys excel at detecting the early stages of deficiencies – thus empowering you to correct small health problems before they become big problems. And symptom surveys can help you to achieve a state of vibrant good health, far beyond the mere absence of disease.

My Nutri-Body® analysis system has become the assessment method of choice by practitioners, for pinpointing nutritional and biochemical weaknesses in their clients. The Nutri-Body® questionnaire includes over 600 questions in 65 categories, the answers to which are analysed by computer.

This book includes 15 symptom surveys excerpted from the Nutri-Body® system, all of which you can easily self-score. I have selected the 15 categories which tend to be most predictive of future health problems.

Yours for the very best of health,
David Rowland

# Listen to Your Body

Long before any disease shows up, changes happen in your body that indicate things are not working as well as they should. These may be pesky little discomforts and inconveniences – things that we take for granted, not realizing that some can be early warning signs of a serious health condition.

Many people have been given a clean bill of health by their doctors, only to drop dead from a heart attack days or weeks later. This is because electrocardiograms can measure problems with the electrical activity of your heart only after they have occurred – and stress tests can indicate problems only after coronary arteries have been at least 70 percent blocked. Neither of these tests are predictive of what could happen in the very near or distant future.

Long before a person experiences a heart attack, however, there are subtle indications that there is plaque progressively building up in the arteries – subclinical symptoms that do not show up on any medical test. Listening to your body's messages in this way could save your life.

Studying the subclinical symptoms presented in this book enables you to predict in which disease direction your body may be headed, if you do not take corrective action. This knowledge empowers you to take pre-emptive nutritional measures to prevent what otherwise could be inevitable.

# Cardiovascular Symptoms

| | |
|---|---|
| | Fingers and/or toes go cold |
| | Arms and/or legs "go to sleep" |
| | Numbness or heaviness in arms or legs |
| | Cramps in hand when writing |
| | Tingling sensation in lips or fingers |
| | Short walk causes cramping or pains in legs |
| | Memory not as good as it used to be |
| | Ankles swell late in the day |
| | Persistent, nagging cough |
| | Breathlessness on exertion, or on lying down |
| | Urinate more than twice during the night |
| | High blood pressure |
| | Impotent or frigid |
| | Chest pain after exertion or emotional stress |

The more of the above symptoms you have – or the more intensely you experience any one of them – the more likely it is that your arteries are in trouble. Fortunately, there is a nutritional program that has a 30-year history of reducing arterial plaque and thereby preventing heart attacks, strokes, and bypass surgery. It is so successful at restoring circulatory flow that it has even reversed many cases of diabetic gangrene, thus saving toes, feet, and legs from amputation. Full details of this arterial cleansing program are explained in my book, *BYPASS THE BYPASS: Restore Circulation Without Surgery*.

The nutritional formula used in the arterial cleansing program is the following. Quantities recommended are per day:

| | |
|---|---|
| Vitamin A | 22,000 to 40,000 I.U. |
| Vitamin D | 40 to 65 I.U. |
| Vitamin C | 4,000 to 4,400 mg. |
| Vitamin E | 600 to 650 I.U. |
| Vitamin B-1 (thiamine) | 66 to 200 mg. |
| Vitamin B-2 (riboflavin) | 30 to 55 mg. |
| Vitamin B-6 (pyridoxine) | 50 to 150 mg. |
| Vitamin B-12` | 160 to 550 mcg. |
| Niacin | 44 to 70 mg. |
| Niacinamide | 20 to 50 mg. |
| Pantothenic Acid | 330 to 550 mg. |
| Folic Acid | 0.4 to 2.2 mg. |
| Biotin | 50 to 122 mg. |
| Choline (bitartrate) | 440 to 725 mg. |
| Inositol | 40 to 55 mg. |
| DL-Methionine | 160 to 550 mg. |
| Magnesium (oxide) | 400 to 555 mg. |
| Potassium (chloride) | 400 to 444 mg. |
| Manganese (gluconate) | 5 to 22 mg. |
| Zinc (gluconate) | 25 to 33 mg. |
| Chromium (chelated) | 130 to 333 mcg. |
| Selenium (chelated) | 200 to 330 mcg. |
| Betaine hydrochloride | 120 to 130 mg. |
| L-Cysteine hydrochloride | 660 to 1,000 mg. |
| Thymus concentrate | 55 to 100 mg. |
| Spleen concentrate | 55 to 100 mg. |
| Adrenal concentrate | 40 to 100 mg. |

Rather than piece together fragmented products, it is more efficient (and cost effective) to take 10 homogeneous tablet per day of a supplement specifically designed for this purpose. Take the tablets in divided amounts with meals (e.g., 4 with breakfast, 3 with lunch, 3 with supper – or 5 with breakfast, 5 with supper). Make sure that your urine turns a bright yellow color (caused by tiny amounts of vitamin C spilling over into the urine). If you do not get this bright yellow color, it means that your digestion is weak and unable to absorb all the nutrients in the tablets – in which case you also need to take supplementary digestive enzymes.

# Pre-Diabetic Symptoms

|  |  |
|---|---|
|  | Pain on inside of left shoulder blade |
|  | Pain on left side of abdomen |
|  | Shingles on trunk of body |
|  | Cold hands or feet |
|  | Feel cold and sweaty |
|  | Shakiness |
|  | Slow healing of cuts, wounds, abrasions |
|  | Constant, intense thirst |
|  | Urinate more than 2 liters (quarts) daily |
|  | Breath smells sweet or of acetone |
|  | Tingling, burning, jabs, or numbness in hands or feet |
|  | Vision failing |
|  | Fainting, blacking out, or convulsions |
|  | Cold sweats of the hands, even when warm |
|  | Complaints relieved by eating, but soon return |
|  | Fainting, blacking out, or convulsions |

If you have any of the above symptoms, you need to consult a physician. If it turns out that you have diabetes, you need to change your diet – to eliminate every form of sugar, and to make sure that you eat mostly protein, complex carbohydrates (e.g., whole grains), and vegetables. You may or may not have to take insulin, however. Some cases of diabetes can be controlled entirely by diet.

The bodies of many people with diabetes do produce enough insulin; however, their cells have become resistant to that insulin. The following nutritional formula reduces insulin resistance.

Daily amounts of nutrients required are **magnesium** (200 mg.), **trimethylglycine** (300 mg.), **zinc** (30 mg.), **alpha-lipoic acid** (200 mg.), **manganese** (15 mg.), **chromium** (200 mcg.), and **vanadium** (300 mcg.).

Diabetics are the highest risk group for cardiovascular diseases. If you are diabetic, regardless of how many boxes you ticked under "Cardiovascular Symptoms", taking the arterial cleansing formula described in that section is a wise precaution, to protect your very vulnerable arteries.

# Prostate Enlargement

|  | |
|---|---|
| | Frequent need to urinate |
| | Reduced force and speed of urination |
| | Difficulty urinating (starting, burning) |
| | Unable to empty bladder completely |
| | Have to urinate more than twice during the night |
| | Back pains associated with urinary difficulties |
| | Discomfort or aching between scrotum and anus |
| | Lost or diminished sex drive |

If you are male and have any of the above symptoms, you need to get a medical diagnosis to rule out prostate cancer. If not cancer, then what you most probably have is an enlarged prostate (benign prostatic hyperplasia) – or BPH for short.

Daily supplementation with the following nutrients has a 25-year history of successfully reducing benign prostatic hyperplasia: **zinc** (75 mg.), **L-alanine** (40 mg.), **glycine** (30 mg.), **glutamic acid** (30 mg.), and **prostate substance** (80 mg.). If some of the above are not available, **saw palmetto** and **pumpkin seed oil** may partially substitute. The zinc, however, is mandatory.

Muscular weakness also contributes to BPH. Prostate muscles need to be exercised, and this can be done by applying gentle finger pressure to the perineum (point midway between scrotum and anus). Hold for two seconds, relax, then repeat five or six times more. Do this twice daily.

# Low Thyroid

| | |
|---|---|
| | Muscles stiff in morning, need to limber up |
| | Fail to feel rested, even after sleeping long hours |
| | Feel "creaky" after sitting still for some time |
| | Heart seems to miss beats or turn "flip flops" |
| | Nauseated in morning |
| | Start slow in morning, gain speed in afternoon |
| | Motion sickness when travelling |
| | Dizzy in morning, or when moving up or down |
| | Sensitivity to cold, prefer warm climate |
| | Hair scanty, dry, brittle, dull, lustreless, lifeless |
| | Hair loss from outer third of eyebrows |
| | Sleeplessness, restlessness, sleep disturbances |
| | Poor short term memory, forgetfulness |
| | Poor response to exercising |
| | Constipation |
| | "Go to pieces" easily, cry easily |
| | Dislike working under pressure or being watched |
| | Gain weight easily, fail to lose on diets |
| | Difficulty concentrating, easily distracted |
| | Yellowish tint to skin on hands or feet |
| | Cracks in bottom of heels |
| | Clogged sinuses |
| | Low pulse rate |
| | Low body temperature, especially at bed rest |
| | Depression |
| | Puffiness of face or eyes |
| | Swelling of hands or ankles |
| | Worse at night: coughing or muscle cramps |
| | FEMALE: Lumpy breasts, cystic breasts |
| | FEMALE: Menstrual irregularity, or excess flow |

The thyroid gland is a gatekeeper. If it produces hormones at a sub-optimal level, then nothing else in the body tends to work well.

Low thyroid function leaves the body vulnerable to acne, allergies, arthritis, asthma, high cholesterol, benign breast disease, cancer, cellulitis, diabetes, eczema, emphysema, gallstones, gout, hives, hypoglycemia, impetigo, infertility, insomnia, lupus erythematosus, mental depression, menstrual irregularities, migraine headaches, obesity, panic attacks, premature aging, sexual dysfunction, tinnitus, toxemia of pregnancy, and urinary tract infections.

If you have only a few of the above symptoms, your thyroid gland may be underactive. If you have many, then it almost certainly is. Blood tests for thyroid hormones are unreliable, because the hormones in the blood may not be getting to the cells and tissues that need them.

Taking your daily temperature tells you more about thyroid performance than blood tests often can. This is because one of the functions of the thyroid is to regulate body temperature. If your thyroid is weak, your temperature will be low.

Take your temperature by mouth three or four times during the day, record the readings, and calculate a daily average. This average should be 37°C (98.6°F) – or slightly higher for women during times of ovulation. Body temperature follows a daily cycle. It may drop slightly during the evening, a little more during sleep, and gradually increase after waking up and moving around. Ideally, body temperature should be 37°C (or slightly above) between the hours of 10 AM and 5 PM. A daily average below 37°C indicates low thyroid function.

Taking the following daily quantities of supplementary nutrients enables a sluggish thyroid gland to shift back into full productivity mode: **Iodine** (4,000 mcg), **L-tyrosine** (300 mg.), **Selenium** (200 mcg.), and **L-cysteine** (500 mg.). This combo is best taken in divided amounts <u>between</u> meals.

Do whatever you need to do to keep your body temperature consistently at 37°C (98.6°F) between the hours of 10 AM and 5 PM, even if it means taking prescription thyroid hormones in addition to the above nutritional formula. (The most natural of the prescription hormones is the generic one called "dessicated thyroid".)

# Adrenal Weakness

| | |
|---|---|
| | Eyes sensitive to bright lights, headlights, sunlight |
| | Tightness or "lump" in throat, hurts under stress |
| | Inability to cope with stressful events |
| | Form gooseflesh easily, or "cold sweats" |
| | Voice rises to a high pitch or is "lost" during stress |
| | Easily shaken up or startled from unexpected noise |
| | Prefer being alone, uneasy when center of attention |
| | Blood pressure fluctuates, sometimes too low |
| | Perfectionist, set high standards |
| | Avoid complaints, try to ignore inconveniences |
| | Work off worries, things left undone cause concern |
| | Allergies (e.g., skin rash, hay fever, asthma, etc.) |
| | Mood swings, tendency to cry easily |
| | Difficulty relaxing |
| | Emotional upsets cause complete exhaustion |
| | Unusual craving for salt |
| | Perspire excessively, sweating of hands or feet |
| | More than usual neck, head, shoulder tension |
| | Blood pressure decreases when standing up |

Adrenal glands in our society tend to be overworked and undernourished. When they become weak or underactive, they leave the body vulnerable to such conditions as chronic fatigue, hypoglycemia, allergies, asthma, diabetes, lowered resistance to infections, low blood pressure, arthritis, dizziness, appetite loss, weight loss, insomnia, and nervousness.

The clinical way to diagnose low adrenal function (hypoadrenia) is the postural blood pressure test. It involves taking blood pressure first while sitting down, and then again when standing up. Under normal circumstances, there should be an increase in the systolic (maximum) blood pressure reading of 4 to 10 mm. Hg. In the standing as compared to the sitting position. If this test does not produce an increase in blood pressure, or if it results in a drop, weak adrenals are the reason.

Daily amounts of nutrients that support adrenal function include **vitamin C** (2,000 mg.), **pantothenic acid** (up to 1,500 mg.), and **vitamin B-12** (1,000 mcg.) – best taken at the same time, in divided amounts with meals. During times of acute stress, depression or grief, the adrenal glands' need for vitamin C soars. In such cases, it is often beneficial to take extra vitamin C to bowel tolerance. This means finding out how much vitamin C it takes to cause either loose stools or excess flatulence, then backing off by one-third. [Example: *If it takes 9,000 mg. of vitamin C to stress the bowels, then 6,000 mg. is the optimal daily amount to take.*]

# Anemia

| | |
|---|---|
| | Pale skin, palms of hand very pale |
| | Fingernails very light in color |
| | Fingernails flat or concave (spoon-shaped) |
| | Thin, fragile, brittle nails |
| | Vertical ridges on nails |
| | Inner side of lower eyelid is pale |
| | Cravings for ice, ice eating |

All the above are symptoms of iron deficiency anemia. This results from a greater demand on stored iron than can be supplied. Red blood cell count may be normal, but there is insufficient hemoglobin, making these cells pale and giving them abnormal shapes. This is probably the most common chronic disease of human kind. It is caused by inadequate iron intake, malabsorption of iron, chronic blood loss, pregnancy and lactation, the destruction of hemoglobin cellular membranes, or a combination of these factors.

Heme is the iron-containing non-protein portion of the hemoglobin molecule, wherein iron is in its ferrous (water soluble) state. Iron found in plant sources is predominantly in its ferric (insoluble) state. This means that the heme iron from animal sources is readily absorbed and utilized by the body, whereas plant sources of iron are not. For this reason, vegetarian diets increase the risk of iron deficiency anemia.

Other nutritional deficiencies are usually involved in anemia, including **vitamin C, iron,** and the **B-complex vitamins,** especially

**B-12** & **folic Acid**. A **hydrochloric acid** deficiency also prevents iron from being absorbed from the diet.

Heme iron is the most utilizable form of iron, and is found only in animal sources (e.g., liver, kidney, heart, red meat, egg yolk, oysters, fish, poultry). Fortunately for vegetarians, there is an exception to this rule. **Ferrous fumarate** is a readily absorbable form of organic iron extracted from plants. Most cases of anemia can be cleared up by taking 30 mg. of iron (from ferrous fumarate) daily, plus a B-complex tablet providing 50 mg. of each of the major B-vitamins and 50 mcg. of each of B-12 and folic acid. [<u>Note</u>: *it takes 100 mg. of ferrous fumarate to provide 33 mg. of elemental iron.*]

# Vitamin C

| | |
|---|---|
| | Skin bruises easily, "black and blue" marks |
| | Hemorrhages or ruptured blood vessels in eyes |
| | Gums bleed easily when brushing teeth |
| | Bluish-red, swollen, or inflamed gums |
| | Loose teeth, loss of dental fillings |
| | Cuts, wounds, or sores heal slowly |
| | Fleeting pains in joints or legs, joint tenderness |
| | Broken capillaries or pink spots on skin |
| | Catch colds, flu, viruses or infections easily |
| | Listlessness, lack of endurance, tire easily |
| | Cuticles tear easily |
| | Excessive hair loss |
| | Restlessness or irritability |
| | Nosebleeds |
| | Bloating or puffiness in face |
| | Anemia |
| | Fragile bones |
| | Thinning or premature aging of skin |

The first eight symptoms on this list are signs of scurvy. We just don't call vitamin C deficiency by that name any more.

We humans (and other primates) suffer from a genetic mutation whereby we do not produce ascorbate (vitamin C) in our livers the way other mammals do. If we could produce vitamin C internally, it would probably be in the range of from 2,000 mg. to 10,000 mg. daily, the higher amounts being required during times of stress.

Contrary to popular misconception, vitamin C produced in the laboratory is every bit as natural as that produced in the livers of mammals. In both cases, glucose is acted upon by the same enzyme, L-gulonolactone oxidase, to produce ascorbate (vitamin C). Dietary supplements containing ascorbic acid or calcium ascorbate provide us with the identical ascorbate molecule that animals produce internally.

# Vitamin B-12

| | |
|---|---|
| | Sore, beefy red tongue |
| | Lemon-yellowish tint to skin |
| | Numbness, tingling, soreness, weakness in hands/feet |
| | Jerking of limbs |
| | Memory loss |
| | Stammering |
| | Apathy, feel as if have lost incentive in life |
| | Depression, moodiness |
| | Hallucinations, delusions |
| | Loss of appetite |
| | Confusion, disorientation |
| | Back pains |
| | Dizziness |
| | Dimmed vision |
| | FEMALE: Menstrual disturbances |

The more symptoms you have on this list, the more likely it is that your body may be heading towards pernicious anemia – a serious condition that if it goes too far can be irreversible, and in some cases can result in heart failure.

Pernicious anemia is an advanced form of vitamin B-12 deficiency. It occurs when the parietal cells of the stomach lining fail to secrete enough intrinsic factor to ensure intestinal absorption of vitamin B-12 (the extrinsic factor). This is due to atrophy of the glandular mucosa of the fundus of the stomach and is associated with a deficiency of hydrochloric acid.

Nutritional treatment involves (a) taking high dose natural **vitamin B-12** (either cyanocobalamin or cobalamin) under the tongue (sublingually), and (b) taking digestive enzyme supplements that provide generous amounts of **hydrochloric acid** (in a stable form, such as betaine hydrochloride). In cases where the nutritional protocol may not be enough, intramuscular injections of vitamin B-12 are required.

Food sources of vitamin B-12 include liver, kidney, muscle meats, fish, cheese, milk products, and eggs. There are no reliable vegetarian sources of this vitamin. Fortunately for vegetarians, supplementary forms of B-12 are extracted from natural bacterial sources.

# Vitamin B-6

| | |
|---|---|
| | Can't remember dreams |
| | Swelling of hands, feet, or ankles (edema) |
| | Unable to close hands into tight, flat fists |
| | Soreness, tenderness, weakness of thumb muscles |
| | Greasy scaliness on skin near nose, mouth, or eyes |
| | Muscular twitching |
| | Greenish tint to urine |
| | Poor co-ordination in walking |
| | FEMALE: Nausea of pregnancy |
| | FEMALE: Acne worse during periods |
| | FEMALE: Swelling of face or abdomen during menses |

The above symptoms all relate to a vitamin B-6 (pyridoxine) deficiency. Number three on the list is carpal tunnel syndrome - in which, in addition to the inability to close one's hand into a tight fist, there can also be numbness, pain, prickling, or tingling affecting some part of the hand (palmar side of the thumb, index finger, radial half of ring finger, radial half of the palm). Most cases of carpal tunnel syndrome can easily be reversed by supplementing with vitamin B-6 and the B-complex vitamins.

B-6 is especially important to women, because this vitamin helps to keep their hormones in balance. Vitamin B-6 not only corrects the nausea of pregnancy and menstrual related edema, it also prevents spontaneous abortion caused by abruptio placenta, the premature detachment of a normally situated placenta after the 20th week of gestation.

23

All the above conditions can be prevented by taking at least 50 mg. of **vitamin B-6** daily (30 times the RDA), in conjunction with similar amounts of the other major B-vitamins (as in a B-50 complex tablet). Therapeutically, it may take 100 mg. per day of B-6 to correct carpal tunnel syndrome.

# Low Stomach Acid

| | |
|---|---|
| | Indigestion, sourness 2 to 3 hours after meals |
| | Abdominal bloating, distension |
| | Full, logy feeling after eating meat |
| | Loss of former taste or craving for meat |
| | Excessive gas, belching, or burping after meals |
| | Burning sensation in stomach, heartburn |
| | Heavy, tired feeling after eating |
| | Constipation |
| | Stools poorly formed, pale, greasy, floating |
| | Undigested food particles in stools |
| | Ridges on fingernails, slow growing nails |

All the above are symptoms of low stomach acid. If the body's production of hydrochloric acid is low, then the entire digestive system is weak – making one vulnerable to such conditions as anemia, pernicious anemia, osteoporosis, and osteoarthritis.

Each link in the digestive chain responds to the one that precedes it. If there is not enough stomach acid, not enough pepsinogen will be converted into pepsin and proteins will not be broken down properly. If the food mass leaving the stomach is not acidified enough by hydrochloric acid, insufficient pancreatic juice and bile will be secreted into the duodenum. Without sufficient bile, globs of fat combine with minerals to form insoluble soaps that cause constipation - and mineral deficiencies. Virtually everyone who is chronically constipated produces insufficient hydrochloric acid

The ideal form of supplementary hydrochloric acid to take is betaine hydrochloride, which comes from beets. Better, however, to support all the interdependent links in the digestive chain. The following is a sample of a digestive enzyme formula that does just that. The amounts given are for a single tablet. You can take one or more tablets with each meal that is difficult to digest: **betaine hydrochloride** (88 mg.), **pepsin** 1:3,000 (110 mg.), **pancreatin** 8X (28 mg.), bile (88 mg.), **bromelain** (44 mg.), **papain** 12M (122 mg.), **peppermint** (66 mg.).

# Hypoglycemia

| | |
|---|---|
| | Irritable if late for a meal or miss a meal |
| | Headaches that are worse after missing a meal |
| | Irritable before breakfast |
| | Easily upset or frustrated |
| | Constant worrying |
| | Fits of anger, agitation, temper outbursts |
| | Episodes of shakiness or tremors |
| | Sudden, strong cravings for sweets or coffee |
| | Episodes of uncontrollable eating, binging |
| | Asthmatic attacks |
| | Anxiety attacks, crying spells |
| | Get hungry soon after eating |
| | Sudden drop in energy in mid-morning or mid-day |
| | Sleepiness after eating, worse if eat dessert |
| | Cold hands or feet |
| | Wake up at night feeling hungry |
| | Wake up in night and can't go back to sleep |
| | Nervousness or headaches relieved by sweets |
| | CHILDREN: Attention deficit or hyperactivity |

Hypoglycemia can be the "you won't like me when I'm hungry" syndrome. The brain is highly dependent on blood sugar (glucose) for its functioning. When blood sugar drops, the brain and central nervous system are affected – often triggering anger, temper outbursts, irritability, anxiety, shakiness, or tremors.

There are two kinds of hypoglycemia. Reactive hypoglycemia is a dip in blood sugar that follows shortly after consuming sugars or sweets. The body overreacts to a sudden increase in glucose by driving it lower than it was before the sugary meal. Anyone with reactive hypoglcyemia needs to practise strict avoidance of foods and beverages that contain any appreciable amount of concentrated sugars of all kinds (e.g., white sugar, brown sugar, raw sugar, cane sugar, corn syrup, maple syrup, honey, molasses, dextrose, glucose, fructose).

Passive hypoglycemia is a response to a gradually diminishing level of blood sugar – which usually depends on how long it has been since the last meal, regardless of what that meal consisted. The hypoglycemic episode could occur anywhere from three to five hours after eating. The solution to passive hypoglycemia is simply to eat five small meals per day rather than the usual three – and to keep non-sugary snacks handy (e.g., nuts, cheese, protein bars).

# Food Allergies

|  | |
|---|---|
|  | Awake in the morning not feeling rested |
|  | An almost "painful" fatigue not helped by rest |
|  | Dark or puffy circles under the eyes |
|  | Spastic colon, colitis, irritable bowel |
|  | Minor, chronic complaints that recur |
|  | High blood pressure |
|  | Bed-wetting, uncontrolled urination |
|  | Insomnia, sleep disturbances |
|  | Heavy sweating not related to exercise |
|  | Fluid retention |
|  | Muscle spasms, aching muscles |
|  | Painful, stiff, or swollen joints |
|  | Depression or crying spells |
|  | Sinus attacks |
|  | Catch colds easily |
|  | History of bronchitis or pneumonia |
|  | Hyperactivity |
|  | Eczema, psoriasis, rashes, dermatitis |
|  | Bladder infections |
|  | Dry stuffy nose, tendency to pick nose |
|  | Bloating or puffiness in face |
|  | Bronchial asthma |
|  | Migraine headaches |

Each of the above symptoms can be caused by a hidden food allergy. So can full blown diseases such as arthritis and colitis. If you or your doctor have been unable to find a cause for any of the above complaints, the good news is that you are probably allergic to something you are eating every day, and by eliminating it you will not only recover but may also prevent a serious disease further down the road. The bad news is that it could be one of your favorite foods that you need to eliminate, and maybe more than one.

Tracking down allergenic foods is not easy. The same symptoms can be caused by different foods in different people. In my book, *NUTRITIONAL SOLUTIONS FOR 88 CONDITIONS*, the chapter entitled "One's Food is Another's Poison" explains how to find the dietary culprits.

If you have allergies of any kind, your adrenal glands probably need some extra help. Daily amounts of nutrients that support adrenal function include **vitamin C** (2,000 mg.), **pantothenic acid** (up to 1,500 mg.), and **vitamin B-12** (1,000 mcg.) – best taken at the same time, in divided amounts with meals.

# Immune Weakness

| | |
|---|---|
| | Chronic colds |
| | Chronic flu |
| | Nasal congestion, sneezing, itching nose |
| | Bronchitis or asthma |
| | Swollen glands in armpit or groin, or tonsillitis |
| | Feeling of puffiness in throat |
| | Soreness on both sides of neck at shoulder level |

The above symptoms are characteristic of viral infections. Viruses are opportunists that take advantage of an immune weakness.

There is an expression, *"You don't catch colds, you eat them."* What this means is that people who catch colds have immune systems that are compromised by hidden food allergies. Antibodies are so battle fatigued from fighting allergenic foods that they are unable to fend off the viral invaders. This happened to me. For the first 30 years of my life, I caught every cold and flu bug going, plus multiple bouts of laryngitis, pharyngitis, bronchitis, and pneumonia. It has been 40 years since I eliminated all the foods to which I was allergic, and in all that time have never caught a single cold or flu bug.

Number one on your anti-viral plan is to identify and eliminate the foods to which you are allergic or intolerant. Number two is to strengthen your immune system during cold and flu season – for which the following daily amounts of supplements are ideal: **vitamin A** (20,000 I.U.), **vitamin C** (3,500 mg.), **methionine** (100 mg.), **thymus** substance (30 mg.), **spleen** substance (30 mg.), and **adrenal** substance (30 mg.)

# Candidiasis

|   |   |
|---|---|
|   | Cravings for sugar, bread, or alcohol |
|   | Indigestion or discomfort after eating fruits or sweets |
|   | Severe reactions to perfume, tobacco, chemicals |
|   | Intolerance to alcohol |
|   | Hypersensitivity to certain foods |
|   | Diarrhea or constipation |
|   | Rectal itching or bladder infections |
|   | Coated or sore tongue |
|   | Chronic sore or scratchy throat, oral thrush |
|   | Feeling of being in a mental fog, "spaciness" |
|   | Tiredness, feelings of being "drained" |
|   | Athlete's foot, toenail or fingernail fungus |
|   | Allergy or sensitivity to airborne molds |
|   | Allergy or sensitivity to moldy or fermented foods |
|   | FEMALE: Premenstrual tension, menstrual cramps |
|   | FEMALE: Endometriosis, uterine fibroids |
|   | FEMALE: Vaginal discharge, burning, itching |
|   | MALE: Prostate problems, impotence |
|   | MALE: Itching of penis or groin |

The above symptoms are typical of an overgrowth of *Candida albicans*, a fungus that is a natural inhabitant of our intestinal tract. Under certain conditions, candida proliferates out of control, forcing itself into the intestinal lining, where it destroys cells in the microvilli, passes into the bloodstream, and invades tissues where it does not belong (i.e., systemic candidiasis).

Many people with candidiasis have been heavy users of broad-spectrum antibiotics, steroid drugs, birth control pills, or alcohol. These drugs destroy the beneficial microflora in the intestines that are the natural antagonists of *C. albicans*.

Most candida programs are not very effective. That is because they do nothing for the cause of the problem. Because *Candida albicans* is a normal inhabitant of our gut, it cannot be starved out of the body. What allows candida to overpopulate is a weak immune system. The only way to reduce the candida population to normal levels is to restore that immunity.

Almost everyone with candidiasis has acquired an allergy to the candida organism. This allergy effectively paralyzes the immune processes that would normally keep the candida in check. This allergy can be reversed, however, simply by taking a homeopathic 30C dilution of *Candida albicans* - 10 drops under the tongue three times daily, between meals. If the only thing one does for candidiasis is to take this homeopathic remedy every day for two months, the candida population will likely be back to normal levels within six months. This time frame can be shortened considerably by also taking garlic and caprylic acid (anti-fungal agents) and *Lactobacillus acidophilus* (or similar probiotic).

If the candidiasis is systemic (i.e., in the bloodstream), then oregano oil will likely be of immediate benefit. Oil of oregano is very potent. It needs to be taken two to three drops under the tongue, twice daily, between meals and at least 30 minutes after taking the homeopathic remedy.

# Premenstrual Syndrome (PMS)

|  |  |
|---|---|
|  | Anxiety, nervous tension, pounding heart |
|  | Irritability, restlessness |
|  | Depression, mood swings |
|  | Emotional outbursts, crying spells |
|  | Headaches, dizziness, fainting |
|  | Backache or cramps |
|  | Insomnia |
|  | Bloating, weight gain |
|  | Forgetfulness, confusion |
|  | Increased appetite or craving for sweets |
|  | Breast tenderness |
|  | Swelling of hands or feet, edema |

The above symptoms are indicative of premenstrual syndrome (PMS) – but only if they occur between 14 days before and 2 days after the menstrual cycle, and at no other time of the month. With the approach of the menses, the extra surge in estrogen levels overtaxes adrenal glands that are only marginally in balance during the rest of the month.

This kind of adrenal weakness makes a woman hypoglcyemic just before her cycle – the reason why she craves sweets and gets irritable only at those times.

The way to banish PMS is to do both of the following, consistently, every day of the month and not just during flareups:

1. Follow a hypoglycemic diet. Strictly avoid foods and beverages that contain any appreciable amount of concentrated sugars of any kind (e.g., white sugar, brown sugar, raw sugar, corn syrup, maple syrup, honey, molasses, dextrose, glucose, fructose).

2. Take the following amounts of adrenal support nutrients daily: **vitamin C** (1,000 mg.), **pantothenic acid** (500 mg.), and **vitamin B-12** (1,000 mcg.) – best taken at the same time, in divided amounts with meals.

# Index to 44 Preventable Conditions

# M

menstrual irregularities, 12
migraine headaches, 12, 29

# N

nausea of pregnancy, 23

# O

osteoarthritis, 25
osteoporosis, 25

# P

pernicious anemia, 21, 25
premenstrual syndrome (PMS), 35
prostate problems, 9, 33
psoriasis, 29

# S

strokes, 3

# U

urinary tract infections, 12
uterine fibroids, 33

# V

vitamin B-6 deficiency, 23
vitamin B-12 deficiency, 21
vitamin C deficiency, 19

# About the Author

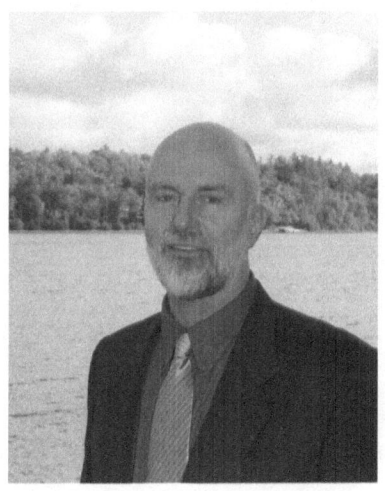

David Rowland is Canada's foremost expert in holistic nutrition. He is publisher of Nutritiapedia®, the free on-line nutritional encyclopedia – and creator of the Nutri-Body® system used by natural health practitioners for determining nutritional and biochemical weaknesses. David founded the Canadian Nutrition Institute (1983), the Nutritional Consultants Organization of Canada (1983), and the Edison Institute of Nutrition (1996). He is also court recognized as an expert in complementary medicine.

Other Books by David Rowland

*ASSESSING BIOCHEMICAL INDIVIDUALITY*

*BYPASS THE BYPASS*
*Restore Circulation Without Surgery*

*NUTRITIONAL SOLUTIONS FOR 88 CONDITIONS*
*Correct the Causes*